Summary, An

(

Amy Myers's

The Thyroid Connection

Why You Feel Tired, Brain-Fogged and Overweight—and How to Get Your Life Back

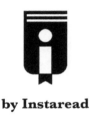

by Instaread

Please Note

This is a summary with analysis.

Table of Contents

Overview

The Thyroid Connection by functional medicine doctor Amy Myers is a self-help book for people who suffer from thyroid dysfunction or suspect that they do. Myers took up her mission to help others understand thyroid conditions when she was in medical school and was diagnosed with Graves' disease, an autoimmune condition that results in hyperthyroidism, or an overactive thyroid. Only after Myers discovered functional medicine, which looks for the root causes of illness rather than treating individual symptoms, did she begin to thrive. Myers used her experience as a patient and doctor to create the Myers Way Thyroid Connection Plan, a 28-day blueprint for restoring health by reducing inflammation; healing digestive problems, such as leaky gut; consuming adequate nutrients; eliminating toxins; adopting stress reduction activities; and using thyroid supplements when needed. Myers advises patients to approach thyroid dysfunction from a holistic perspective so they can put an end to difficult symptoms and begin to thrive.

The thyroid is vitally important to health because it provides fuel for every cell in the body and plays a critical role in hormone production. It is an integral part of a larger system, which includes the hypothalamus, the part of the brain that governs hunger, thirst, metabolism, and hormone production; and the pituitary gland, which manages growth, reproduction, and the production of thyroid-stimulating hormone (TSH). The varied symptoms of an overactive "hyperthyroid" and underactive "hypothyroid" or "dysfunctional thyroid" include weight loss, weight gain, brain fog, depression, anxiety, sluggishness, and hair loss. Most thyroid conditions are the result of an autoimmune disorder in which a person's immune system is so taxed that it begins fighting against itself.

Unfortunately, thyroid conditions are often not properly diagnosed or identified. Conventional medical doctors use a wide range of thyroid hormone levels for measuring thyroid function, and what they consider normal isn't necessarily optimal. When a condition is diagnosed, traditional physicians tend to overlook remedies like diet and lifestyle intervention in favor of prescription drugs and invasive procedures—treatments designed to address the effects of thyroid malfunction but not the underlying cause.

People suffering from thyroid conditions can learn to take charge of their health by educating themselves about the nature of thyroid problems, asking their doctor for a full panel of tests, and making important changes to their diet and overall lifestyle. This way, they can support their body in healing and performing at its maximum capacity.

The Thyroid Connection was published by Little, Brown on September 27, 2016, and became an instant *New York Times* bestseller.

Important People

Amy Myers is a medical doctor certified in functional medicine by the Institute of Functional Medicine, of which she has been a member since 2010. She is the author of the *New York Times* bestseller *The Autoimmune Solution* (2015).

Key Takeaways

1. A functional medicine approach to treating thyroid dysfunction is based on the idea that patients can play a vital role in supporting their own health.

2. Thyroid problems are often overlooked in conventional medicine.

3. The thyroid, which is located in the neck, is part of a chain of systems that create hormones.

4. Functional medicine is customized and considers a number of ways that the thyroid could be malfunctioning.

5. Thyroid problems are usually the result of an autoimmune disorder.

6. Finding the right dosage and type of hormone supplement can make a huge difference in a person's overall health.

7. There are many factors that lead to hyperthyroidism or hypothyroidism.

8. Nutrients play a vital role in proper thyroid function.

9. Stress reduction is essential to proper thyroid function.

Thank you for purchasing this Instaread book

**Download the Instaread mobile app to get
unlimited text & audio summaries
of bestselling books.**

Visit Instaread.co
to learn more.

Analysis

Key Takeaway 1

A functional medicine approach to treating thyroid dysfunction is based on the idea that patients can play a vital role in supporting their own health.

Analysis

Conventional medicine operates from the philosophy that some symptoms—such as stress, diminished energy, and lack of sex drive—are a natural result of aging. Doctors tell patients they should take appropriate medication but otherwise learn to live with their compromised health. In contrast, functional medicine operates under the assumption that patients at any age—and with any condition including thyroid problems—can thrive by making important lifestyle changes, such as eating foods that support thyroid and immune system functioning, and lowering their stress levels.

The benefits of taking a holistic approach to treating disease are numerous and can be applied to conditions other than thyroid disease. For example, in her 2016 book *A Mind of Your Own,* Dr. Kelly Brogan describes how she was practicing as a traditional psychiatrist when she was diagnosed with Hashimoto's thyroiditis, an autoimmune disease that caused hypothyroidism. Her immune system began attacking her thyroid tissue, which resulted in inflammation and an underperforming thyroid. Brogan, who was in her early thirties, had always lived a high-stress lifestyle and had "suboptimal dietary habits"—which meant she liked fast food. Her doctors offered her a prescription and told her that she'd be on medication for this chronic condition for the rest of her life. This was unacceptable to Brogan, who had otherwise been healthy her whole life and who knew that drugs often come with a host of side effects. In an effort to avoid lifelong medication, Brogan started researching alternatives and eventually reversed her condition with healthy foods, exercise, and meditation. Brogan soon realized that she could help her own patients who were suffering from dysregulated thyroid and manifesting depression and anxiety, simply by recommending the same lifestyle interventions. Now Brogan has a thriving practice in which she teaches her patients how to make interventions so that they can live in a state of vibrant health without prescription drugs. [1]

Key Takeaway 2

Thyroid problems are often overlooked in conventional medicine.

Analysis

Approximately 27 million Americans have been diagnosed with thyroid dysfunction, but there are likely millions more cases that are ignored by doctors. This is because symptoms of thyroid problems are common ailments, such as depression, weight gain or loss, achy muscles and joints, disrupted sleep patterns, and fatigue. If patients' test results show them to be within a normal thyroid range, doctors are less likely to pinpoint a compromised thyroid as the cause because they might be looking at an incomplete set of data. Men in particular are less likely to be tested for thyroid problems.

Author Ian Probert is one such example. He has Hashimoto's thyroiditis, but it took 15 years for him to get a proper diagnosis. In isolation, his symptoms were relatively common, so he thought he was depressed. He felt listless and unable to concentrate. He gained a lot of weight. He says, "My brain was lost in a deep fog, life was percolating away from me. I was slowly—very slowly—dying." Probert began fainting on a regular basis. He suffered from a string of colds and had a hip injury that never healed in addition to frequent bouts of psoriasis. Only when a friend asked him if he'd had his thyroid checked did Probert go in for testing. He learned than the level of TSH in his body—which indicates thyroid dysfunction—was at 99, far beyond the normal range of 0.5-4.5 milli-international units per liter (mIU/L). He began taking medication which has mostly alleviated his problems including the brain fog and weight gain. He was able to get back to his writing profession and rarely has incidents of depression. By writing about his experience, Probert aims to help others who are suffering but may not know the thyroid might be the source of their problems. [2]

Key Takeaway 3

The thyroid, which is located in the neck, is part of a chain of systems that create hormones.

Analysis

The thyroid system starts in the hypothalamus, which receives signals about thyroid hormone levels in the blood. If levels are low, the hypothalamus sends a signal to the pituitary gland, which then releases TSH to signal to the thyroid to release hormones to the blood.

Many people lack knowledge about the thyroid and how it works in concert with other systems, which leads to the conception of the thyroid as a "mysterious" organ. [3] As she tried to diagnose her own thyroid condition, writer Olga Khazan realized that there's a lot of fuzzy information about how the gland performs. She observes, "Every other yoga class I attend involves some pose 'that's good for the thyroid.'" [4] Khazan learned about the experience of Dana Trentini, a woman who started a popular blog about treating the thyroid with unconventional methods. Trentini's blog has upwards of 1.6 million page views per month, and she has nearly 250,000 followers on her Facebook page, which is evidence of the unmet demand for information about thyroid conditions. Trentini's struggle with thyroid dysfunction came about when she miscarried because she and her doctors didn't recognize the extent of her thyroid problems. Trentini told Khazan, "I could feel that I was very ill, but I was the kind of person who believed doctor knows best. I should have gotten a second or third opinion. I should have done something, but I didn't. The blog began because I was angry with myself." [5]

Khazan's and Trentini's experiences are somewhat understandable because it takes nearly two decades for scientific research to reach doctors, who then influence the general public's understanding. As recently as 2009, researchers were attempting to understand the significance of the "hypothalamus-pituitary-thyroid axis" by looking at critically ill patients and how their available levels of T3, the active form of thyroid hormone, played a role in their illness. [6] While they found that critically ill patients had a "disturbance" in the hypothalamus-pituitary-thyroid axis, researchers still found the role that low T3 played somewhat mysterious. [7]

Key Takeaway 4

Functional medicine is customized and considers a number of ways that the thyroid could be malfunctioning.

Analysis

Patients should be evaluated based on their individual needs. Often, conventional doctors aren't looking at the right information. For example, a traditional doctor might see normal levels of thyroid hormones T3 and T4 in a patient's blood and neglect to measure how much of those hormones are free, or available to enter the cells, in the case of T3, or to be converted to T3, as in the case of T4. By contrast, functional medicine calls for a comprehensive analysis of thyroid function and how it affects a patient.

This is a point of frustration for conventional doctors. Dr. David Cooper, who teaches endocrinology at Johns Hopkins School of Medicine, notes that he is sometimes pressured to look at and treat the thyroid and says it comes from "angry patients who feel doctors don't listen to them." [8] However, these patients are responding to a general lack of insight into thyroid malfunction displayed by many conventional doctors.

Key Takeaway 5

Thyroid problems are usually the result of an autoimmune disorder.

Analysis

Thyroid-related autoimmune problems are characterized by the immune system attacking the thyroid. Autoimmune problems can develop in numerous ways, but the cause is the same: the immune system has become overtaxed and is no longer able to tell the difference between foreign substances and organic matter, such as thyroid tissue. Once people develop one autoimmune disease, their risk of developing subsequent autoimmune diseases is high.

For example, a young woman who is facing the stress of two critically ill parents who live overseas might be burdening her immune system in ways she doesn't even realize—until she gets a diagnosis of Hashimoto's thyroiditis. Despite her own health problems, she might decide it's necessary to leave her job and go care for her parents, a move that makes her susceptible to developing further illnesses because of the stress she experiences by moving abroad. At the very least, being her parents' full-time caretaker will not support her healing from Hashimoto's because of the physical and emotional challenges of caring for declining parents. She might then develop aching joints and be diagnosed with rheumatoid arthritis, another autoimmune disorder. Because her immune system has become compromised, she doesn't have the physical strength her body requires to ward off further immune system disorders. The resulting avalanche of symptoms might lead to difficulty in diagnosis and treatment because the numerous symptoms could mask the root cause of her problems.

Key Takeaway 6

Finding the right dosage and type of hormone supplement can make a huge difference in a person's overall health.

Analysis

Every person responds differently to medication. For example, a woman with hypothyroidism might receive a supplemental thyroid medication that boosts her T3 and T4 levels but react with increased anxiety because her body chemistry is very sensitive to T3. However, depending on how well a person responds to diet and lifestyle changes, a supplement might not be necessary at all.

In recent years, alternative thyroid supplements have become more widely available. Dr. Victor Bernet, the chair of endocrinology at the Mayo Clinic in Jacksonville, Florida, realized the power of natural supplements when test results for one of his patients showed a remarkable improvement in thyroid hormone levels, a development Bernet called "inexplicable." [9] The patient told him that a friend had given him a supplement intended to treat "low energy," which led Bernet to investigate further. [10] In 2014, Bernet and a team of researchers published findings from a study that tested 10 nonprescription thyroid boosters. They discovered that nine of these contained T3 and T4 hormone levels higher than prescription drugs. [11] One in particular contained 91 micrograms of T4, an amount that far exceeds the standard amount of 25 micrograms. These findings suggest that it's imperative for people taking supplements to receive regular checks. As Bernet explains, "Thyroid hormone has a narrow therapeutic window…it's easy to go over or under [the optimal dosages]." [12]

Key Takeaway 7

There are many factors that lead to hyperthyroidism or hypothyroidism.

Analysis

The complex thyroid system can become compromised in many ways. For example, a person can be exposed to environmental toxicity that results in reverse T3, a thyroid hormone that takes up space and inhibits normal T3 from attaching to cells. Fluctuations in sex hormones can have a disruptive effect on the thyroid. Additionally, having a permeable intestinal wall can trigger an immune response; the more often this happens, the more taxed the immune system becomes and the more likely a person will develop an autoimmune disorder that will affect the thyroid.

Writer Meghan O'Rourke, who suffers from Hashimoto's, describes her experience attempting to determine the root of her physical symptoms, including sluggishness. When she finally received her diagnosis, she thought her symptoms would be relieved simply by following her doctor's recommendations. But six weeks later, she wasn't feeling any better. She returned to her doctor, who suggested raising the dosage of her supplemental hormone and casually mentioned that some of her patients improve when they cut out wheat from their diets. O'Rourke remarks, "I began to suspect that whatever was wrong with me wasn't going to be as clear-cut as a germ or a malfunctioning organ." [13] She had family members who suffered from autoimmune disorders including Hashimoto's, ulcerative colitis, and rheumatoid arthritis. O'Rourke learned from her aunt that these conditions were all related. Desperate to feel better, she began looking online and fell into a maze of blogs by fellow sufferers. She heeded the overwhelming advice to change her diet drastically and, although it took some time, eventually she began to feel better. The process of gaining control was not without struggle. She writes, "To be sick in this way is to have the unpleasant feeling that you are impersonating yourself." [14] O'Rourke's experience indicates the very intricate nature of human biology.

Key Takeaway 8

Nutrients play a vital role in proper thyroid function.

Analysis

To produce optimal levels of T3 and T4, people need to consume protein so that the body can produce tyrosine, which, along with iodine, is essential for thyroid hormone formation. Other nutrients, such as iron and selenium, are required to help the body turn stored T4 into active T3.

Recent scientific findings confirm the importance of nutrients in correcting and reversing thyroid conditions. In 2016, researchers reviewed 16 controlled studies that examined the role of selenium supplements in lowering the amount of serum thyroid peroxidase, or thyroid antibodies, which indicate an autoimmune thyroid response. [15] In another 2016 study, researchers looked at levels of iron and iodine to see how they correlated with thyroid function in more than 200 Nepalese children ages 6-12. They found that children with iron and iodine deficiencies—a common problem in Nepal—had thyroids that functioned at suboptimal levels. [16]

Key Takeaway 9

Stress reduction is essential to proper thyroid function.

Analysis

The sympathetic nervous system helps a person react immediately to physical and emotional stress, and the parasympathetic nervous system helps a person relax and recover from such responses. When a person is in a sustained state of stress, the body struggles to produce the proper amount of cortisol, a stress hormone. Because cortisol production is governed by the hypothalamus and the pituitary gland, the production of thyroid hormones is also disrupted.

Fortunately, there are many ways to reduce stress, such as meditation, yoga, and hot baths. Recently, researchers found that attending live music concerts can reduce cortisol levels. In a partnership between the Royal College of Music and Imperial College London, scientists studied 117 subjects who attended two concerts of music by composer Eric Whitacre. They found that all subjects had lowered levels of cortisol and cortisone, both of which are glucocorticoids that play a role in stress response. [17] This study marks the first published evidence of a cultural event having an effect on the endocrine system. Daisy Fancourt, the lead researcher, says, "It is of note that none of these biological changes were associated with age, musical experience or familiarity with the music being performed. This suggests there is a universal response to concert attendance among audience members." [18] The findings indicate that the effect of the music works on a biological level regardless of demographic and other factors.

Another unique relaxation response has been associated with casual gaming. In 2015, scientists at Embry-Riddle Aeronautical University revealed findings from a study that compared casual gaming as a stress reducer to a more traditional method of guided meditation and sitting in stillness. Researchers found that casual gaming was actually more beneficial in promoting stress reduction and a positive mood than traditional meditation. [19]

Author's Style

Amy Myers writes passionately and knowledgeably about helping others navigate the confusing landscape of thyroid dysfunction. She shares her personal experience living with an autoimmune thyroid condition and emphasizes the need for patients to take full and total control of their own health in areas including diet and exercise. She tells the stories of patients who have benefited from her functional medicine approach.

Myers's writing about the thyroid and how it functions within the larger biological system is clear, accessible, and practical. She uses metaphors to explain why different parts of the body react under certain conditions and is detailed in her clinical explanations. She devotes a substantial part of the book to explaining how doctors can mistreat or fail to diagnose thyroid problems. Myers offers an exhaustive strategy for helping people become educated about all aspects of the thyroid so that they can most effectively partner with their doctors. For example, she includes information on which tests to request and what insurance companies generally cover. She provides specific information about the myriad supplements, both natural and synthetic, so that people have a fuller understanding of how these supplements can assist their recovery.

Myers also outlines the Myers Way Thyroid Connection Plan, which includes an easy-to-follow regimen aimed at calming inflammation, healing the gut, harnessing the curative powers of natural foods, removing toxins from the home, treating infections that may be exacerbating an immune response, and reducing stress. She lists healthy recipes and provides information so that readers can have a tailored approach to taking supplements. She offers suggestions for ways to reduce stress, such as steam room sessions. The text contains lists of available resources, such as the Myers Online Community, where people suffering from thyroid problems can connect directly with one another to share information and find support. It also contains links to further reading on tracking symptoms, planning for meals, and other topics. Appendices include information on writing a letter to the doctor, creating a mold-free environment, and doing a home detox.

Author's Perspective

Amy Myers was in medical school when she began having a strange collection of physical symptoms including anxiety, sudden weight loss, and tremors. Her doctors dismissed her condition as stress, but deep down, she knew that something was wrong. After she pressed her doctor to run more tests, Myers was diagnosed with Graves' disease, an autoimmune condition that results in hyperthyroidism. She was frustrated by her doctor's recommendations: to take medicine, or have a procedure that would destroy her thyroid by injecting iodine and obliterate its function, or have it surgically removed altogether. Myers sought alternative means to heal her condition. She has been treating patients with the Myers Way Thyroid Connection Plan for 10 years. Myers is a former Peace Corps volunteer. Her current work as a physician and best-selling author is an extension of her desire to be of service to others.

~~~~ END OF INSTAREAD ~~~~

Thank you for purchasing this Instaread book

**Download the Instaread mobile app to get
unlimited text & audio summaries
of bestselling books.**

Visit Instaread.co
to learn more.

References

1. Brogan, Kelly, and Kristin Loberg. *A Mind of Your Own: The Truth About Depression and How Women Can Heal Their Bodies to Reclaim Their Lives.* New York: Harper Wave, 2016, p. 86.

2. Probert, Ian. "My underactive thyroid was slowly killing me." *The Guardian.* September 8, 2013. Accessed October 14, 2016. https://www.theguardian.com/lifeandstyle/2013/sep/08/underactive-thyroid-was-slowly-killing-me

3. Khazan, Olga. "Sleepy, Stressed, or Sick? Why thyroid diseases are so common—and so mysterious." *The Atlantic Monthly.* February 9, 2015. Accessed October 14, 2016. http://www.theatlantic.com/health/archive/2015/02/why-is-one-of-the-most-common-diseases-still-so-mysterious/385256/

4. Ibid.

5. Ibid.

6. Mebis, L., and G. van den Berghe. "The hypothalamus-pituitary-thyroid axis in critical illness." *The Netherlands Journal of Medicine.* 67:10 (November 2009):332-340. https://www.ncbi.nlm.nih.gov/pubmed/19915227

7. Ibid.

8. Khazan, Olga. "Sleepy, Stressed, or Sick?"

9. Rabin, Roni Caryn. "Thyroid Supplements with a Kick." *The New York Times.* January 20, 2014. Accessed October 14, 2016. http://www.nytimes. com/glogin?URI=http%3A%2F%2Fwell.blogs. nytimes.com%2F2014%2F01%2F20%2Fthy-roid-supplements-with-a-kick%2F%3F_r%3D0

10. Ibid.

11. Kang, Grace Y., et al. "Thyroxine and Triiodothyronine Content in Commercially Available Thyroid Health Supplements." *Thyroid* 23:10 (September 2013): 1233-1237. http:// online.liebertpub.com/doi/abs/10.1089/ thy.2013.0101?journalCode=thy&

12. Rabin, Roni Caryn. "Thyroid Supplements."

13. O'Rourke, Meghan. "What's Wrong With Me?" *The New Yorker.* August 26, 2013. Accessed October 14, 2016. http://www.newyorker.com/ magazine/2013/08/26/whats-wrong-with-me

14. Ibid.

15. Wichman, Johanna, et al. "Selenium supplementation significantly reduces thyroid autoantibody levels in patients with chronic autoimmune thyroiditis: A systematic review and meta-analysis." *Thyroid* October 2016.

Accessed October 14, 2016. http://online.liebertpub.com/doi/pdf/10.1089/thy.2016.0256

16. Gelal, Saroj Khatiwadasanta, et al. "Association between iron status and thyroid function in Nepalese children." *Thyroid Research* 9:2 (2016). http://search.proquest.com/openview/77393a38b37a69c7ec2b5816f2f117b-c/1?pq-origsite=gscholar&cbl=55245

17. Fancourt, Daisy, and Aaron Williamon. "Attending a concert reduces glucocorticoids, progesterone and the cortisol/DHEA ratio." *Public Health* 132 (February 2016): 101-104. http://www.publichealthjrnl.com/article/S0033-3506(15)00499-0/abstract

18. Boult, Adam. "Attending live music events 'reduces your stress hormones'—study." *The Telegraph*. April 12, 2016. Accessed October 14, 2016. http://www.telegraph.co.uk/science/2016/04/12/attending-live-music-events-reduces-your-levels-of-stress-hormon/

19. Russoniello, Carmen, et al. "The effectiveness of casual video games in improving mood and decreasing stress." *Journal of Cybertherapy & Rehabilitation*. 2:1 (Spring 2009) 53-66. Accessed October 26, 2016. https://www.researchgate.net/publication/289131468_The_effectiveness_of_casual_video_games_in_improving_mood_and_decreasing_stress

Lightning Source UK Ltd.
Milton Keynes UK
UKHW02f0618060718
325319UK00011B/408/P